THIS BOOK

BELONGS TO

....

....

Thank you for Purchasing my book and taking the time to read it from front to back. I am always grateful when a reader chooses my work and I hope you enjoyed it!

With the vast selection available online, I am touched that you chose to be purchasing my work and take valuable time out of your life to read it. My hope is that you feel you made the right decision.

I very much would like to know what you thought of the book. Please take the time to write an honest and informative review on Amazon.com. Your experience and opinions will be of great benefit to me and those readers looking to make an informed choice.

With much thanks.

Table of Contents

INTRODUCTION

What Exactly is Cortisol?

Cortisol, a glucocorticoid hormone produced by your adrenal glands, is then released into your body.
Hormones are compounds that interact through your blood with your organs, skin, muscles, and other tissues to coordinate different biological actions. These signals tell your body what to do and when to do it.

Glucocorticoids are a kind of steroid hormone. They control your muscle, fat, liver, and bone metabolism while lowering inflammation in all of your bodily parts. Glucocorticoids have an effect on the sleep-wake cycle as well. Your two small, triangular-shaped adrenal glands, known as suprarenal glands, are located on top of your two kidneys. They are found in your body's endocrine system.

- Cortisol, a vital hormone, affects every organ and tissue in your body. It regulates a number of critical tasks, including the response of your body to stress.

- helping to regulate your body's metabolism, which is how it consumes fats, proteins, and carbohydrates.

- Blood pressure control while decreasing inflammation

- Blood sugar regulation

- Aiding in the regulation of your sleep-wake cycle

Your body regularly monitors your cortisol levels to ensure they remain steady (homeostasis). ***Cortisol levels that are higher or lower than usual might be harmful to your health.***

Is Cortisol a Stress Hormone?

Cortisol is often referred to as the "stress hormone." It has various additional key effects and functions throughout your body in addition to directing your body's stress response.

Furthermore, bear in mind that, from a medical standpoint, there are numerous forms of stress, including:

Rapid anxiety When you are abruptly and momentarily under danger, you feel acute stress. Scenarios that cause acute stress include barely avoiding a car accident or being followed by an animal.

Chronic (long-term) stress is caused by ongoing events that cause you to feel irritated or nervous. Chronic stress may be caused by a variety of factors, including a difficult or time-consuming job or a long-term illness.

- **Traumatic stress disorder:** Traumatic stress arises when you experience a life-threatening event that leaves you feeling terrified and helpless. Experiencing a war, a sexual assault, or a catastrophic meteorological event such as a tornado may all cause traumatic stress. These occurrences may occasionally lead to post-traumatic stress disorder (PTSD).

Cortisol is produced by your body in response to any of these types of stress.

HOW DOES CORTISOL AFFECT YOUR BODY?

All of your body's tissues include glucocorticoid receptors. Cortisol may therefore have an effect on almost all organ systems inside the body, including the;

- Neurological system.
- Defense system.
- Circulatory system.
- Respiratory apparatus.

- Reproductive apparatus (male and female).
- Muscles and bones.
- System of vegetation (skin, hair, nails, glands and nerves).

Cortisol, in further detail, has the following impacts on your body:

- **Taking control of your body's stress response:** When you are stressed, your body may generate cortisol after releasing "fight or flight" hormones like adrenaline, which puts you on high alert. Furthermore, cortisol drives your liver to manufacture glucose (sugar) for rapid energy during stressful periods.

- **Metabolism regulation:** Cortisol helps to regulate how your body uses carbohydrates, proteins, and fats for energy. reducing inflammation Cortisol may strengthen your immunity momentarily by lowering inflammation. However, if your cortisol levels are consistently high, your body may get used to having too much of it in your blood, causing inflammation and impairing your immune system. Blood pressure management Uncertainty surrounds the specific mechanism through which cortisol regulates blood pressure in humans. High cortisol levels, on the other hand, may cause high blood pressure, while low cortisol levels can cause low blood pressure.

- **Increasing and controlling blood sugar:** Cortisol normally balances the effects of insulin, a hormone produced by the pancreas to manage your blood sugar. While insulin lowers blood sugar, cortisol raises it by releasing glucose stored in the body. Chronically higher cortisol levels may lead to high blood sugar levels (hyperglycemia). ***This might lead to type 2 diabetes.***

- **Controlling your sleep-wake cycle:** Cortisol levels are typically lowest in the evening before going to sleep and highest in the morning immediately before waking up. This demonstrates that cortisol is vital for the onset of wakefulness and influences your body's circadian rhythm.

Healthy cortisol levels are required for life and the maintenance of various physiological systems. If your cortisol levels are consistently too high or too low, your overall health may suffer.

How Does Your Body Manage Cortisol Levels?

The production of cortisol in your adrenal glands is controlled by your pituitary gland, a tiny gland located underneath your brain, and your hypothalamus, a small part of your brain involved in hormone regulation. When your blood cortisol levels fall, your hypothalamus releases corticotropin-releasing hormone (CRH), which signals your pituitary gland to produce adrenocorticotropic hormone (ACTH). ACTH then stimulates your adrenal glands to produce and release cortisol.

For your body to have optimal levels of cortisol, your brain, pituitary, and adrenal glands must all be functioning properly.

Medical practitioners may test your cortisol levels using blood, urine, or saliva. They will choose the best test for you based on your symptoms.

WHAT LEVEL OF CORTISOL IS CONSIDERED NORMAL?

Cortisol levels in your blood, urine, and saliva normally peak in the morning, decline over the day, and reach their lowest around midnight. This schedule may change if you work a night shift and sleep at different times throughout the day.

The normal ranges for the majority of tests that measure cortisol levels in your blood are as follows:

- Between 6 and 8 a.m., take 10 to 20 micrograms per deciliter (mcg/dL).
- At 4 p.m., levels ranged from 3 to 10 mcg/dL.

Normal ranges might vary from lab to lab and from person to person. If you need a cortisol level test, your healthcare practitioner will review the results and advise you if additional testing is required.

WHAT CAUSES HIGH CORTISOL LEVELS?

Hypercortisolism, or the extended presence of abnormally high cortisol levels, is sometimes misdiagnosed as **Cushing's syndrome**, a rare disorder. Cushing's syndrome and excessive cortisol levels may be caused by: using large doses of corticosteroid medicines to treat other conditions, such as prednisone, prednisolone, or dexamethasone. **Tumors** that produce **adrenocorticotropic hormone (ACTH).** They are usually found in your pituitary gland. Neuroendocrine tumors in other organs, such as the lungs, may sometimes raise cortisol levels.

Adrenal hyperplasia, or tumors of the adrenal glands, cause an excess of cortisol production.

The severity of your Cushing's syndrome symptoms is determined by your cortisol levels. The following are common symptoms and warning indications of increased cortisol levels:

- Gaining weight, especially around the face and stomach.
- Fatty deposits between your shoulder blades.
- Wide purple stretch marks on the abdomen (belly).
- You have weak muscles in your thighs and upper arms.
- High blood sugar levels often lead to Type 2 diabetes.
- High blood pressure (hypertension).
- Hair growth that is excessive (hirsutism) in those who are born with a gender preference.
- Fractures and brittle bones (osteoporosis).

What Causes Low Cortisol Levels?

Hypocortisolism, or lower-than-normal cortisol levels, is a symptom of adrenal insufficiency. There are two types of adrenal insufficiency: primary and secondary. Adrenal insufficiency may be caused by:

- The major cause of adrenal insufficiency An autoimmune reaction, in which your immune system unjustifiably destroys healthy cells in your adrenal glands, is the most common cause of primary adrenal insufficiency. Addison's disease is the medical term for this condition. A lack of circulation to the tissues or an infection might both injure your adrenal glands (adrenal hemorrhage). All of these factors limit cortisol production.

- Adrenal secondary insufficiency: A pituitary tumor or an underactive pituitary gland (hypopituitarism) may inhibit ACTH production. Because ACTH signals your adrenal glands to make cortisol, a low ACTH level also indicates a low cortisol level.

Furthermore, if you stop using corticosteroid medicines suddenly after a lengthy period of use, you may have lower than normal cortisol levels.

What Symptoms Point to Low Cortisol Levels?

- Fatigue is a symptom of adrenal insufficiency, which results in lower-than-normal cortisol levels.
- Weight loss that was not intended
- Slow digestion
- Lower blood pressure (hypotension).

How can I reduce my cortisol levels?

If you have Cushing's syndrome, you will need medical treatment to reduce your cortisol levels (very high levels). The majority of treatments need either medication or surgery. In addition, if your cortisol levels are low, you should seek medical assistance.

There are, however, a variety of regular steps you may take to try to lower your cortisol levels and keep them within safe ranges, such as:

- **Get enough sleep:** Cortisol levels that are too high have been connected to persistent sleep issues such obstructive sleep apnea, insomnia, and working the night shift.
- **Regular physical activity:** Numerous studies have indicated that regular exercise improves sleep quality and decreases stress, both of which may reduce cortisol levels gradually.

- **Control your stress levels and negative thinking patterns by learning to:** Being aware of your breathing, heart rate, and other signs of tension may help you spot stress and prevent it from worsening.

- **Improve your deep breathing skills by doing the following:** Controlled breathing stimulates the parasympathetic nervous system, which decreases cortisol levels.

- **Take it easy and chuckle:** When you laugh, endorphins are produced, and cortisol is lowered. Hobbies and fun hobbies may make you feel better, which may help lower your cortisol levels.

- **Maintain positive relationships:** Relationships play an important part in our lives. Cortisol levels may rise, and frequent stress may be caused by unfriendly and unpleasant encounters with family members or coworkers.

CHAPTER 1:

Reduce Cortisol Levels Quickly and Effectively

Understanding the different cortisol levels can help you select which ones you should always aim for.

It is always important to maintain your mental wellness. Stress and anxiety may have a negative impact on your physical and mental health.

Cortisol, widely known as the stress hormone, is produced by the adrenal glands. When we are stressed or worried, it rises, and when we are calm, it falls. When cortisol levels rise, the body directs all of its resources into coping with the stressor rather than managing other internal functions such as the immune and digestive systems.

I like to imagine myself being hunted by a lion. Whether a lion is following you, you don't care if you become ill or need to use the restroom. Cortisol normally aids in the control of weight, appetite, body metabolism, blood pressure, and glucose; however, when under prolonged stress, you may also experience pre-diabetes, weight gain, insomnia, increased anxiety or depression, headaches, memory issues, brain fog, digestive problems, and other symptoms.

However, I recognize that regulating anxiety is easier said than done, so I've supplied you with a variety of tactics to help you lower cortisol levels and have a level head during this volatile time in our lives. Furthermore, these are lifestyle changes that you can do for the rest of your life rather than pandemic-specific recommendations;

- **Consume a plant-based, whole-food diet.** A bad diet consisting of processed foods and added sugars can raise cortisol levels, increasing your risk of diabetes and high blood pressure. Consume plenty of fiber; fruits and vegetables are good sources. Fiber aids in hormone balance by modulating hormones and intestinal bacteria. Diet is really important; it accounts for 80% of the battle.

- **As needed, provide vitamins.** A well-balanced diet should always come first, and supplements should always be used under the direction of a doctor. However, magnesium, which helps to regulate cortisol levels, is the most important mineral we use in our therapeutic practice when it is recommended. Vitamin B12, folic acid, and vitamin C may also help in cortisol metabolism.

- **Take a deep breath.** Numerous studies show the benefits of doing deep breathing exercises three to five times every day for at least five minutes. According to studies, it helps to decrease cortisol levels, reduce anxiety and depression, and improve memory. To begin, use a deep breathing app such as Insight Timer or Calm.

- **Limit your caffeine intake.** Adrenal fatigue, also known as chronic stress exhaustion, is a condition in which the body's cortisol levels are out of whack. They get so tired by it that they often rely on coffee to get them through the day. When the caffeine wears off, they get tired again. Caffeine may raise cortisol levels without addressing the underlying problem of hormone balance.

- **Get adequate sleep.** For the body to recover, we need at least seven to eight hours of sleep every night. Despite its importance, it often slips by the wayside because of our busy schedules. Regular physical activity The American College of Lifestyle Medicine suggests 30 to 50 minutes of exercise every day. And walking your dog doesn't count; you should be pushed to the point where you can chat to someone while working out but can't sing.

- **Make a diary entry.** It might be beneficial to jot down thoughts on paper at times. If they are happy thoughts, you can revisit them; if they are unpleasant, you can cleanse them so you don't think about them all the time.

- **Have fun with your hobbies.** Playing an instrument, drawing, crafts, or gardening are all delightful hobbies that may take your mind off stressful thoughts and events. Step outdoors. Being among plants, trees, flowers, birds, and other living things may assist to calm the mind. If possible, take a walk around the block before relaxing on your front porch. When the weather heats up, it will be easier to take breaks and spend time outdoors.

- **Be a fearless leader.** Making fear the priority might be perplexing. It allows us to do things that would otherwise be wrong or imprudent. You may lead positively by being aware, taking deep breaths, and following the suggestions given above.

I appreciate that it may seem overwhelming, but you are not required to apply all of this advice at once. Making modest, good changes is the best way to obtain long-term outcomes. Introduce one or two at a time until they become second nature, then gradually add more. Someone who travels slowly and steadily frequently wins the race.

What Happens When Cortisol Levels are Elevated?

Over the past 20 years, research has shown that moderate to high cortisol levels may lead to a range of health issues, including

- Chronic disease If your cortisol levels are consistently raised, you are more likely to develop high blood pressure, heart disease, type 2 diabetes, osteoporosis, and other chronic illnesses.

- Putting on weight Cortisol may increase hunger and signal the body to switch metabolism to fat storage.

- Weariness and difficulty sleeping It may interact with sleep hormones, influencing the amount and quality of sleep.

- Concentrating problems Some people have trouble focusing and a lack of mental clarity, which is commonly referred to as "brain fog."

- Dysfunction of the immune system Cortisol excess may impair the immune system, making it more difficult to fight infections.

- Cushing's syndrome Cushing's syndrome is an uncommon but fatal illness caused by very high cortisol levels.

- Excessive activity or malignancy of the pituitary or adrenal glands, chronic stress, and pharmacological adverse effects are all possible causes of increased cortisol levels (e.g., prednisone, hormonal therapy)

Furthermore, pre-existing chronic disease (such as obesity) may increase cortisol levels, resulting in a "chicken or the egg" scenario.
It is thus essential to consult with a skilled health practitioner to establish the underlying reason for your health problems. You may also want to begin some effective lifestyle changes that will assist you in better controlling your cortisol levels. Here are a few recommendations:

1. **Make sure you get adequate sleep.**

Making sleep a major priority may aid in lowering cortisol levels. Cortisol levels that are too high have been related to persistent sleep issues such obstructive sleep apnea, insomnia, and shift work.

One study of 28 shift workers found that those who slept during the day (night shift employees) rather than at night (day shift employees) had higher cortisol levels.

Rotating shift workers have been linked to worse health outcomes such as type 2 diabetes, heart disease, obesity, and mental health problems. Furthermore, the word "insomnia" refers to the inability to sleep. Numerous variables, including stress and obstructive sleep apnea, may play a role. This may result in greater levels of cortisol in the blood, which may affect your daily hormone cycles, energy level, and other aspects of your health.

Although you may not have complete control over your sleeping pattern, whether you work the night shift or a rotating shift, there are numerous steps you may take to improve your sleep.

- **Create a nightly routine.** Establishing a consistent nightly routine, such as taking a shower or reading a book, may tell your body and brain to begin preparing for sleep.

- **Every day, establish a regular bedtime and wake-up time.** A regular sleep schedule has been shown to be one of the greatest approaches for improving sleep.

- **Exercise first thing in the morning.** Regular exercise may improve your sleep quality, but it should be done at least 2-3 hours before bed.

- **Consume less coffee.** Avoid caffeine-containing meals and drinks six hours or more before going to bed.

- **Stay away from alcohol and nicotine.** Both medications have an effect on the duration and quality of sleep.

- **Limit your exposure to strong light at night.** 45-60 minutes before going to bed, reduce your exposure to strong and/or blue light. Instead of reaching for your phone, try reading a book or listening to a podcast in bed.

- **Sleep in a quiet location.** Reduce distractions by using white noise, earplugs, and phone quiet.

- **Having a nap.** If your sleep time is limited due to shift work, napping may help you feel less drowsy and prevent having a sleep deficit. Naps, on the other hand, may impair the sleep of non-shift workers.

2. <u>Get some exercise, but not too much</u>

"Depending on the intensity, exercise may either boost or lower cortisol levels."

Cortisol levels rise quickly after vigorous exercise, but then fall a few hours later. This rapid surge assists in synchronizing the body's growth in preparation for the challenge. Furthermore, frequent exercise minimizes the quantity of cortisol released.
Numerous studies have shown that regular exercise may assist with improved sleep, stress reduction, and overall well being, all of which can help reduce cortisol levels over time.

It's worth noting that regular exercise has been related to enhanced tolerance to acute stress and may reduce the negative health effects of stress, such as raised cortisol levels.

Going overboard, on the other hand, might have the opposite effect. Set a weekly target of 150-200 minutes of largely low- to moderate-intensity exercise and allow for recovery time in between sessions. Cortisol, a stress hormone, is released by the adrenal glands. It helps your body cope with stressful situations because your brain releases it through the sympathetic nervous system, sometimes known as the "fight or flight" system, in response to a range of sources of stress.

While cortisol production may assist in your capacity to avoid danger in the short term, when levels are overly high for a long length of time, this hormone may potentially do more damage than good. This may lead to a variety of health issues, such as weight gain, high blood pressure, diabetes, heart disease, difficulty sleeping, mood changes, and low energy.

It is thus essential to consult with a skilled health practitioner to establish the underlying reason for your health problems. You may also want to begin some effective lifestyle changes that will assist you in better controlling your cortisol levels. Here are a few recommendations:

3. <u>Learn to recognize troubling ideas.</u>

Paying attention to your worried thoughts may help you to reduce them. The key to mindfulness-based stress reduction is being more aware of your own stress-inducing thoughts, accepting them without resistance or judgment, and allowing yourself the space to process them. You may detect stress early on by teaching yourself to be aware of your breathing, thoughts, pulse rate, and other tension-related indicators.

You may avoid being a victim of your worried thoughts by focusing your attention on being aware of your emotional and physical state. Being aware of stressful thoughts allows you to form an intentional reaction to them. A study involving 43 women in a mindfulness-based program, for example, discovered a link between the ability to express and explain stress and a lower cortisol response.

Lower cortisol levels have also been seen in other studies after regular mindfulness meditation.

Consider adding mindfulness-based techniques into your daily routine for better stress management and decreased cortisol levels.

4. **<u>Exhale</u>**

Deep breathing is a simple stress-reduction technique that may be done anywhere. Controlled breathing, like mindfulness-based practices, promotes the parasympathetic nervous system, sometimes known as the **rest and digest** system, which decreases cortisol levels.

Deep breathing is a popular practice in mindfulness-based disciplines such as meditation and yoga which put a strong emphasis on breathing and the mind-body connection and have been shown in studies to lower participants' cortisol levels. Numerous studies have shown that these approaches may help lower cortisol and stress.

5. **<u>Have fun and laugh.</u>**

Having fun and laughing also aids in the reduction of cortisol levels. When we laugh, endorphins are produced, while stress hormones like cortisol are inhibited. It has also been linked to better mood, less stress and pain perception, lower blood pressure, and a stronger immune system. It's worth noting that both real and forced laughter may relieve stress.

It has been shown, for example, that laughing yoga, a kind of yoga that stimulates purposeful bursts of laughter, decreases cortisol levels, lowers stress, enhances mood, and increases perceived vitality.

Having interests may also boost feelings of well-being, resulting in lower cortisol levels. Gardening had a bigger effect on lowering levels than typical occupational therapy, according to a study of 49 middle-aged veterans.

Another study including 1,399 individuals found that those who engaged in activities they enjoyed had lower cortisol levels.

Furthermore, relaxing music may reduce cortisol levels.

6. <u>Maintain positive connections</u>

Friends and family may provide both immense happiness and terrible strain. Cortisol levels show the dynamics of this.

Cortisol is present in minute amounts in your hair. The concentrations of cortisol discovered along a hair's length signify cortisol levels throughout the time that specific section of the hair was forming. Because of this, researchers can estimate levels over time.

According to a research on conflict styles in 88 couples, nonjudgmental mindfulness was associated with a faster recovery of cortisol to normal levels after an argument. As a consequence, expressing compassion and understanding to your partner and receiving it in return may aid with cortisol regulation.

Support from loved ones may also help reduce cortisol levels while under stress. One study, for example, discovered that connecting lovingly **verbally or physically** with a romantic partner or platonic friend before doing a challenging activity lowered stress-related markers such as heart rate and blood pressure.

7. <u>Take care of a pet</u>

Having animal companions in your life may lower your cortisol levels. In one study, children who engaged with a therapy dog during a brief session saw lower levels of anxiety and cortisol.

Another study involving 48 people discovered that talking to a dog was more soothing than seeking advice from a friend in a socially difficult situation.

In a third study, the efficacy of dog companionship to reduce cortisol levels was compared between pet owners and non-owners.

Because the latter group had already benefited from their animals' company at the start of the study, they experienced a greater drop in cortisol when they were given canine companions.

Because of the well-known benefits of pets for decreasing stress, many long-term care facilities and university/college campuses have introduced pet therapy as a natural cortisol- and stress-reducing activity.

8. <u>Eat a well-balanced diet.</u>

Nutrition may have a positive or negative impact on cortisol levels. While all meals should be consumed in moderation, paying attention to what you eat may assist you in better controlling your cortisol levels and reducing the impacts of stress.

Consuming a lot of added sugar on a regular basis may cause your cortisol levels to increase. It's worth noting that a high-sugar diet may limit cortisol synthesis under stressful conditions, making it more difficult for your body to manage. A diet strong in added sugar, refined carbohydrates, and saturated fat may result in considerably higher cortisol levels when compared to a diet high in whole grains, fruits, vegetables, and polyunsaturated fats.

A healthy gut microbiome, which refers to all of the bacteria that live there, has been related to greater mental health in multiple studies. As a consequence, consuming foods that improve gut health may reduce stress and anxiety while also improving overall health.

These extra meals may help you reduce your cortisol levels:

- **Chocolate** that is bitter Dark chocolate's strong flavonoid content has been shown to lower cortisol synthesis by the adrenal glands' response to stress. complete grains Whole grains have more fiber and plant-based polyphenols than processed grains, which may aid with stress and digestive health.

- **legumes and lentils.** They are high in fiber, which helps digestive health and controls blood sugar levels. Whole fruits and vegetables Whole fruits and vegetables are high in antioxidants and polyphenolic compounds, which aid to protect cells from free radicals.

- **Tea with herbs L-theanine**, a relaxing chemical present in green tea, has been linked to reduced stress and better mental clarity. Both prebiotics and probiotics are available. Yogurt, sauerkraut, and kimchi may include friendlier, symbiotic bacteria. Prebiotics like soluble fiber feed these microorganisms. Probiotics and prebiotics have been linked to improved gastrointestinal and mental health.

- **Nourishing fats Diets** high in unsaturated fat and low in saturated fat are associated with improved physical and mental health. Omega-3 fatty acids, in particular, are strongly linked to stress reduction and brain function. Excellent sources include nuts, seeds, and fatty seafood. Water. It is therefore even more important to keep hydrated throughout the day, since dehydration has been linked to a temporary increase in cortisol levels.

9. <u>Take particular vitamins</u>

In addition to a nutrient-rich diet, several supplements may help lower cortisol levels.

Fish oil is an excellent source of omega-3 fatty acids, which are thought to reduce cortisol levels.

When compared to a placebo in a 3-week randomized controlled trial, supplementation with both docosahexaenoic acid (252 mg/day) and fish oil (60 mg/day) significantly lowered cortisol levels in response to a stressful task. Another study of 2,724 people found that those with greater blood levels of omega-3 fatty acids had lower levels of cortisol and inflammation.

Even though fish is a rich source of omega-3s, you may want to supplement with fish oil. Check with a medical professional first to be sure it's right for you.

CHAPTER 2:

Cortisol Hangover

According to some estimates, anxiety during a hangover affects around 12% of people, and the degree varies depending on the person.

When the body recovers from a night of drinking, it experiences physiological stress, which causes a hangover. When the body is under stress, such as from a sickness or an accident, physiological stress typically develops. A hangover has comparable symptoms. In addition to affecting our immune system, it elevates cortisol levels, generally known as the "stress hormone," blood pressure, and heart rate, all of which are altered by anxiety.

Changes occur in the brain as well. Dopamine, a neurotransmitter, is less active in the brain during a hangover, according to study. This is essential since dopamine significantly affects anxiety. Due to the heightened tension that comes with a hangover, it may be difficult to manage any additional stress that emerges during the day.

It's intriguing that stress and lack of sleep, which might mirror the symptoms of a hangover, can induce mood and cognitive performance declines (including attention and memory). Because of weariness, stress, and other unpleasant hangover symptoms, daily tasks may be difficult to complete. A person suffering from a hangover, for example, may be too preoccupied with controlling their nausea, headache, or exhaustion to adequately handle troubling thoughts.

According to studies, people's emotions shift adversely when they have a hangover. Furthermore, numerous people reported they felt less able to manage their emotions while they were drunk. In other words, people experience unpleasant sentiments and have a difficult time getting back up after a hangover.

Another study looked at the effect of hangovers on executive performance (mental skills which are important for many aspects of our daily life, including working memory, flexible thinking and self control). Participants' cognitive skills were tested by assigning them a range of tasks, such as memorizing a string of letters and remembering it when requested.

Individuals who were hungover performed badly on important executive function tasks. Executive processes enable us to suppress worried thoughts and cope with concern. It may help to understand why some people sense anxiety when they are inebriated if their cognitive capacities are hindered.

Almost all hangovers are accompanied by some kind of discomfort, such as a headache or muscle aches. However, studies have found that those who "catastrophize" their pain—that is, exaggerate it or anticipate the worst—are more likely to suffer from anxiety. According to study, this group is more prone to severe hangovers. This may assist to explain why some people suffer from anxiety while others do not.

Those who are inclined to anxiety may be more susceptible to hangxiety. Negative life events, drinking-related sorrow or wrath, drinking-related guilt, and even specific personality traits (such as neuroticism) have all been connected to hangover mood swings. Even people who profess to be very shy had higher levels of hangxiety, which may be associated with indicators of alcohol use disorder.

Together, these aspects demonstrate how hangxiety varies from person to person and why it is a major part of hangovers. Aside from being unpleasant, mood changes caused by a hangover have been linked to excessive drinking, increased interpersonal conflict, and lower workplace efficiency.

The same techniques that assist with anxiety will also aid with hangxiety. Mindfulness techniques, meditation, and general self-care may be included. Allowing yourself the following day to recover and avoiding other pressures (such as work or family concerns) prior to your night out may help you manage with the extra psychological burden.

Some people even use a hangover to reconnect with one another, discussing their previous drinking session and even dealing with their problems together. Of course, refraining from alcohol totally or drinking minimally is the best way to avoid getting hangxiety.

How to Get Over a Psychological Hangover

If you've ever had too much to drink, you know what a hangover is and how tough it is to get rid of one. Nausea, sluggishness, and dizziness are the most frequent alcohol hangover symptoms. True, a night of drinking might leave you feeling unpleasant the next day. Did you know that a time of acute emotional overload, in addition to drinking, may have the same consequences as a hangover? The emotional hangover is a real thing.

The bulk of the time, emotional hangovers are caused by catastrophic occurrences or prolonged stressful periods. A loved one's death, a breakup with a spouse or friend, a job loss, an accident, or receiving bad medical news may all trigger stress. Some people may have this hangover effect even after small confrontations, such as an argument with a close friend or a difficult day at work. A lengthy day of forced engagement may result in an emotional hangover for introverts.

If you are now experiencing a great deal of emotional upheaval, this is the perfect book for you. We'll go through eight practical techniques for dealing with an emotional hangover.

1. <u>Eat Healthfully</u>

Coffee, sweets, and chocolate, for example, have a reputation for inducing anxiety and exacerbating emotional hangovers. Consume as many fruits and leafy greens as you can afford, since they will improve both your physical and emotional health. Many people make the mistake of attempting to relax by drinking their concerns away in the expectation that it would make them feel better, but this just makes their emotional problems worse. *When you're suffering from an emotional hangover, you don't want to disrupt your brain's chemical equilibrium.* You must consume a variety of nutritious foods in order for your sensitive mind to recover after a stressful period.

2. <u>Seek Compassion</u>

Unhealthy social ties are often the cause of negative energy. It's conceivable that your parents dislike you without reason, that racism is common in your line of work, or that your boss is sexist. If not dealt with promptly, this negativity may easily develop into an emotional hangover. Instead of pushing your anger inside your chest, speak with a trustworthy friend or counselor. The training of a life coach may also help you stop the loop of exhausting negativity and erroneous thinking and reintroduce you to the cycle of optimism. Enrolling in this course or working with a life coach will help you break free from your never-ending cycle of sadness and emotional hangover.

3. <u>Research and Reflect</u>

Meditation helps you avoid recalling painful experiences from the past by moving you outside of your thoughts. It allows you to focus on your breathing and take in the tranquility all around you. Reading inspiring literature may also help you relax.

4. **Drink Plenty of Water**

Anger and sadness may be draining. You shed a lot of tears and sweat while struggling to handle all of the difficult emotions that pervade your existence. You should drink lots of water to replace your fluids.

5. **Rest**

When you have an emotional hangover, particularly after a traumatic encounter that physically drains your body, do nothing. Perhaps you put in too much effort on a job assignment, and then your boss took all the credit. Perhaps you should sleep.

6. **Exercise**

Physical exercise has several mental health benefits, including reduced anxiety and depression. Yoga, dancing, biking, or going for a walk may all boost your mood.

7. **Spend time with those you care about.**

Perhaps you made a mistake, but beating yourself up over it will not help. Pay a visit to a friend or family member. Anyone who is understanding and uncritical is acceptable. Spend time with them, get their feedback, and solicit new ideas from them. It is therapeutic to be in the company of your loved ones.

8. **Go on a nature stroll.**

Give a tree a hug. Examine the surface with your bare feet. Dance in the rain. Enjoy the blooms. Your indoor garden requires care. Take a walk. You have a rock in your hand. Get immersed in nature's unspoiled splendor. Breathe in some fresh air. Being in nature is the best remedy for emotional hangovers.

Cortisol is advantageous when taken correctly and at the right times. However, if cortisol and sleep deprivation are not regulated, you may find yourself trapped in a vicious cycle.

When you think about cortisol, the first thing that comes to mind is how closely it is tied to stress? which is why it is known as **"*the stress hormone.*"** While cortisol may be your best buddy when you're rushing to catch a bus or make a deadline, few people are aware of its considerable impact on sleep. If you've ever had difficulties falling or staying asleep all night, your body may be overstimulated by this stress hormone.

In any event, cortisol is necessary for everyday functioning. This hormone is necessary not only for inducing the fight-or-flight response, but also for waking us up in the morning and lowering physiological inflammation (when cortisol is present in normal amounts). Only an untimely, consistent infusion of cortisol into your body may disrupt your sleep patterns, as well as your short- and long-term health and wellbeing.

Do High Cortisol Levels Have an Impact on Sleep Quality?

When your body is constantly stressed, it is compelled to stay in the fight-or-flight mode, which contributes to chronic stress. After a threat has passed, your stress response system generally shuts down. A common example would be a hectic lifestyle that is overburdened with responsibilities to family, employment, and leisure time.

As you may anticipate, this leads to imbalanced cortisol production as the HPA axis goes haywire. Instead of the usual peaks and troughs, your cortisol cycle is now fixed on high cortisol release. While high cortisol levels may help you get through the day, having too much cortisol throughout the day or too close to night might disrupt your sleep-wake cycle.

Other indications of excessive cortisol levels include mood changes, fast weight gain, and high blood pressure. An overabundance of this stress hormone also jeopardizes sleep quality. Because stress causes the production of adrenaline and noradrenaline, which boosts your body temperature and heart rate. As a consequence, falling asleep will be more difficult, as will transitioning from light to deep sleep.

HPA axis hyperactivity alters your usual sleep architecture in the following ways:

- Increased sleep fragmentation (nighttime awakenings)

- There is a decrease in slow-wave sleep and restorative sleep.

- Shorter sleep length and insufficient sleep

- Insomnia is caused by too much cortisol, which raises your sleep debt and diminishes your vigor the next day. You're obviously not feeling or performing at your best. It becomes worse since there is a link between specific sleep issues and HPA axis function. For example, obstructive sleep apnea and insomnia may both be caused by HPA axis activation.

- Sleep deprivation raises cortisol levels.

While too much cortisol causes sleep problems, a lack of sleep elevates cortisol levels in your body. If you don't get enough sleep, your body won't have time to slow down cortisol production, resulting in increased levels of the stress hormone throughout the day.

In other words, you're too aroused to sleep, and your bedtime is later than usual. You are now trapped in a vicious cycle of increased cortisol and little sleep, which is detrimental to your everyday functioning and overall well-being.

However, cortisol excess is caused by more than just a lack of sleep. Even if you have met your sleep requirements, an inconsistent sleep pattern that is not in sync with your internal clock may cause your cortisol cycle to become erratic. .

How can I lower my cortisol levels and sleep better?

While it's easy to become trapped in the nightmare labyrinth of cortisol overstimulation and sleep loss, effective sleep hygiene may help you get out of it by keeping your sleep debt low and your circadian rhythm in good operating condition. As a result, reduced sleep debt and circadian alignment promote a healthy homeostatic system that maintains your body's cortisol levels within an optimal range. When cortisol levels are normal, your sleep-wake cycle returns to normal (together with all other important hormones).

CHAPTER 3:

Cortisol and Weight Reduction

Cortisol is dubbed the "stress hormone" for good reason. When we are under a lot of stress, our cortisol levels rise, which helps us stay alert for an attack or escape a danger.

Long-term stress, on the other hand, may elevate cortisol levels. It becomes a problem when we are constantly overloaded and in a condition of fight or flight as a result of urgent work deadlines, family obligations, or financial problems. Lack of sleep and inconsistent sleeping patterns can raise stress hormone levels. When cortisol levels are often elevated, you may begin to gain weight.

One of the key activities of cortisol is:

- prompting your fight-or-flight response to keep you vigilant When levels are high in the early morning, they wake you up. Controlling your metabolism and how your body uses protein, fats, and carbohydrates for energy Control of the immune system and decrease of inflammation

Cortisol is therefore not the enemy since it is required for everyday function. It runs on a 24-hour cycle called the circadian rhythm. Cortisol levels rise early in the morning and aid in waking up. Then, as the day progresses, it progressively falls until it reaches its lowest point about midnight before gradually rising again. It increases again early in the morning, and the cycle continues.

When everything is working correctly, this cortisol rhythm ensures that your body generates the necessary quantities of cortisol at the appropriate times throughout the day.

The timing of this cortisol cycle is determined by your chronotype, which is your proclivity to sleep and wake up at various times throughout the day. If you're a night owl, for example, your cortisol peak will be later in the morning. Your overall cortisol levels will also be reduced.

Cortisol levels rise beyond the morning high when we are in fight-or-flight mode. However, it usually returns to normal after whatever was generating your anxiety has passed. Cortisol levels, on the other hand, remain elevated when you are continually in flight-or-fight mode and under a lot of stress.

An overabundance of cortisol may cause anything from insomnia to mood swings, weight gain, and cardiac issues.

Be aware that Cushing's syndrome causes the body to create an excess of cortisol. It may be caused by the use of steroid medications, a pituitary gland tumor, an adrenal gland tumor, or both.

How Does Cortisol Affect Weight Gain?

Obesity and weight gain are linked to elevated cortisol levels, especially in the abdomen region. When exposed to stressful situations, individuals who were thicker around the midsection emitted considerably more cortisol, according to one study.

But what happens behind the scenes?

You've probably experienced the feeling of stress eating. When we're overloaded at work, we feel the urge to go for a bag of chips or a bar (or two) of chocolate to help us get through our growing to-do list. Cortisol levels may play a role in part of this stress-eating tendency.

According to one study, persons who had strong cortisol responses when exposed to stressful situations ate more calories than those who had low cortisol reactions. Furthermore, those with high cortisol levels ate a lot more sweet foods throughout the day. As a result, even being stressed may encourage you to want unhealthy foods and consume more in general.

Cortisol may influence appetite-regulating hormones such as leptin, the hormone that makes you feel full, but the specific mechanism by which it causes overeating is uncertain.

When your cortisol levels are high, your body is triggered to release glucose that has been stored in the liver, causing your blood sugar levels to rise. This is useful when you need a burst of energy to run for the bus, for example.

If your blood sugar levels are persistently high, you risk acquiring obesity and insulin resistance. Furthermore, excess glucose that the body cannot use as energy may be stored as fat, especially belly fat, resulting in weight gain.

When your cortisol levels are consistently raised, it is more difficult to sleep, and this may lead you to gain weight. High cortisol levels make it harder to fall asleep, cause you to wake up more often at night, and reduce the amount of time you sleep.

This makes getting the amount of sleep you need, which is determined by your genetic makeup, much more challenging. When you don't get enough sleep, you have less energy to exercise, less self-control to stick to a diet, and your hunger hormones are thrown out of sync, all of which may lead to overeating.

The occasional cortisol rise caused by a stressful situation is not harmful. Persistent stress, on the other hand, and the accompanying consistently increased cortisol levels, are not.

Reduce your cortisol levels by using stress-reduction measures such as:

- Exercising, but not excessively or recently

- Regular exercise is an excellent way to reduce stress and improve your overall well-being. It may also reduce your cortisol's response to stress, and low-intensity exercise actually reduces cortisol levels.

- Cortisol levels increase during high-intensity exercise because your body is under stress. While this is occasionally OK, if you over-exercise, you may suffer the harmful consequences of excess cortisol.

- Make sure you workout at the right time and don't overdo it. Prevent exercising too close to bedtime to avoid interrupting your sleep, which may lead to increased cortisol and weight gain.

- Maintaining a Low Sleep Debt Sleep deprivation is one of the most stressful things you can do to your body. It may raise your evening cortisol levels by 37% to 45%, leading to weight gain and greater sleep deprivation. Furthermore, lack of sleep has been linked to weight gain, making it easy to get into a vicious cycle.

Another decreasing trend? Not only can lack of sleep induce worry, but anxiety may also cause insomnia. Both may lead to weight gain. You may avoid all of this by knowing your sleep requirements and attempting to satisfy them every night.

Stress causes cortisol levels to increase, resulting in weight gain. However, many of us are unaware of the harmful impact that circadian misalignment and considerable sleep debt have on the body. Everyday activities, such as exercise or a cup of coffee, may have an effect on cortisol levels. Reduce your stress, regulate your coffee and exercise consumption, get adequate sleep, and live in tune with your circadian clock to break the cortisol weight gain loop.

CHAPTER 4:

What is the Connection Between Sleep and Weight?

Adequate sleep, as well as sleep at the optimal periods for your circadian cycle, are both necessary for weight loss.

While the majority of us blame the fat epidemic in our modern society on poor eating habits and a lack of regular exercise, there is one element that is sometimes overlooked: lack of sleep. After a bad night's sleep, you won't have the energy to go to the gym, and it will be tough to resist those doughnuts. However, the association between sleep and weight loss is more complicated than that.

Sleep deprivation may have an impact on your metabolism, capacity to reduce weight, and hunger hormones. Furthermore, your weight loss efforts may succeed or fail if you do not get enough sleep at the appropriate times for your biological clock.

It would be much easier to maintain a healthy weight if you can improve your sleep and sleep pattern. However, if you get them wrong, you may wind up gaining weight as well as having difficulty reducing it.

How Sleep can Possibly Affect Weight Loss

Sleep and weight have a direct relationship. Here's how a bad night's sleep impacts your waistline.

- Sleep deprivation causes you to eat more unhealthy foods.

If you don't get enough sleep, your appetite hormones are out of balance. As a consequence, the hormones ghrelin, which induces hunger, and leptin, which produces fullness, drop. As a consequence, your appetite will increase, causing you to consume more.

> - Losing sleep impairs your ability to govern yourself, making it more difficult to resist high-calorie, high-carbohydrate junk food. Your endocannabinoid system, which regulates your appetite and reward regions in your brain, is also stimulated, which increases your hunger for particular meals.

Sleep deprivation also has an impact on how well your brain's hypothalamus region operates, which is important for managing your appetite and regulating how much energy you consume.

> - The last element is that if you are awake for a longer amount of time, you have more opportunity to eat. Despite the fact that being active burns more calories than sleeping, being up for an extended length of time improves your chances of ingesting more calories than you expend.

This is supported by science. Adults may eat an extra 385 calories each day after a night of insufficient sleep, according to study.

Short sleepers, those who receive less than five hours of sleep each night, are more likely to gain weight, according to a research analysis on sleep and obesity. And it doesn't take much to boost their odds.

According to the research, missing only one hour of sleep each day was associated with a 0.35 kg/m2 rise in body mass index (BMI).

However, we all react differently to sleep deprivation. Everyone needs a varied amount of sleep each night. It is inherited in the same way as height and eye color are, and not everyone gets eight hours.

According to one research, the recommended amount of sleep each night is 8 hours 40 minutes, plus or minus 10 minutes, although 13.5% of people may need 9 hours or more.

• Caloric Burn is Reduced by Sleep Deprivation

Sleep deprivation lowers your energy levels and motivation, making it more difficult to participate in physical activity and calorie-burning activities like going for a run or going to the gym.

Aside from exercise, sleeping less naturally reduces your calorie consumption. Following five nights of four hours of sleep, studies have revealed that your resting metabolic rate, which accounts for the bulk of the calories you burn each day, is much lower.

As a consequence, sleep deprivation increases calorie intake while decreasing calorie expenditure, resulting in weight gain.

• Sleep Deprivation Has an Impact on Glucose Metabolism

Even if you aren't eating more calories, having less sleep causes your body to store more fat.

According to study, those who sleep for less than 6.5 hours each night produce 50% more insulin and have 40% worse insulin sensitivity than those who get an average amount of sleep (defined as getting 7.5 to 8.5 hours a night).

Insulin resistance may develop as a consequence of high insulin levels, increasing your risk of type 2 diabetes and obesity. When your body develops insulin resistance, you can't absorb glucose as easily. If you have too much glucose in your blood, it may be stored as fat in the body (especially around the belly) if it isn't used as fuel.

• Sleep deprivation undermines other weight loss attempts.

As a result, sleep deprivation may impede other weight-loss attempts in addition to increasing calorie consumption, calorie burn, and body fat storage.

One study, for example, looked at overweight people who were subjected to calorie restriction for two weeks while getting either 8.5 or 5.5 hours of sleep each night. You're undoubtedly aware of who lost the most weight. Those who slept for 8.5 hours lost more body weight and were less hungry than those who slept for 5.5 hours.

"A lack of proper sleep may impede the efficacy of typical food therapy for weight loss," the researchers concluded in their study.

To make the most of your diet and calorie-cutting efforts, you must also attend to your sleep requirements.

What Effect Does Belly Fat Have on Sleep?

If you're trying to lose weight, you'll probably want to lower your belly fat as well. And both are linked to lack of sleep.

Obesity and abdominal obesity have both been linked to sleeping five hours or less each day. In addition, frequent six-hour sleepers had higher BMIs, fat percentages, and abdominal circumferences than regular seven- to eight-hour sleepers.

Furthermore, a 2022 study found that those who slept for just four hours each night for 14 nights consumed more calories, gained more weight, and grew more belly fat than the control group, including visceral fat (fat that surrounds the organs) and subcutaneous fat.

Sleep deprivation elevates your body's level of the stress hormone cortisol, and excessive cortisol levels may cause your body to accumulate fat, especially around the belly. Sleep deprivation may also lead to insulin resistance, which raises your chance of developing type 2 diabetes and leads your body to accumulate excess fat around, you guessed it, your belly. But it's not just about how much sleep you get. Obesity and abdominal obesity have been linked to poor sleep efficiency, which is defined as being up for a significant amount of the night.

Maintaining a low sleep debt reduces the risk that higher ghrelin, insulin, and cortisol from sleep deprivation may lead to weight gain. You'll also have more resolve to stick to your diet and more energy to work out. Individuals who regularly slept 6.5 hours per night were able to reduce their caloric intake by 270 calories per day by sleeping an extra 1.2 hours each night, according to a 2022 research. This would equal to a 26-pound weight loss over the course of three years.

Many people struggle to find ways to dramatically reduce their calorie intake in order to lose weight, but just getting more sleep may help.

• Sleep is an important aspect of weight loss.

A definite correlation exists between getting adequate sleep and decreasing weight. Sleep deprivation has an impact on everything from hunger hormones to fat storage, which may lead to binge eating, weight gain, and belly fat. Even while dieting, it might be tough to avoid unhealthy foods and find the will to exercise. However, sleep hygiene is seldom addressed in diet regimens.

However, in addition to getting enough sleep, you also need time to sleep around your circadian cycle.

Maintaining a low sleep debt and living in rhythm with your circadian cycle might help you avoid weight gain, make weight reduction easier, and keep the pounds off once you've lost them.

CHAPTER 5:

Stress, Menopause, Infertility, and Cortisol

A stressful situation, whether environmental, such as an imminent work deadline, or psychological, such as chronic job loss concern, may kick off a chain reaction of stress hormones, resulting in well-timed physiological changes. A stressful incident may cause the heart to beat and the breathing to quicken. Perspiration beads develop when muscles contract.

This complex of stress reactions is referred to as the "fight-or-flight" response because it was established as a survival strategy to enable humans and other organisms adapt quickly to potentially lethal conditions. Because of the well-timed, yet virtually instantaneous, sequence of hormonal changes and physiological responses, someone may reject the assault or flee to safety. Unfortunately, stressors such as traffic, work pressure, and family concerns may all trigger the body to respond.

Researchers learned about the long-term effects of chronic stress on physical and psychological health over time, as well as how and why these responses occur. Activating the stress response repeatedly wears down the body over time. According to studies, chronic stress raises blood pressure, promotes the formation of artery-clogging deposits, and changes the brain in ways that may lead to anxiety, depression, and addiction. More preliminary evidence suggests that chronic stress may also contribute to obesity, either directly (by causing people to eat more) or indirectly (by causing them to move more) (decreasing sleep and exercise).

The stress response begins in the brain. When a person is presented with an oncoming automobile or another threat via the eyes, ears, or both, the amygdala, a part of the brain that assists in emotion processing, gets information. The amygdala interprets the images and sounds. When it senses danger, it instantly sends a distress signal to the hypothalamus.

When a stressful event happens, the amygdala, a region of the brain involved in emotion processing, sends a distress signal to the hypothalamus. This portion of the brain works as a command center for the nervous system, which interacts with the rest of the body to equip the person with the power to fight or flee. In some respects, the hypothalamus resembles a command post. This part of the brain connects with the rest of the body through the autonomic nervous system, which governs automatic physical activities such as breathing, blood pressure, heartbeat, and the expansion or contraction of vital blood arteries and small airways in the lungs known as bronchioles. The autonomic nervous system is made up of two parts: **the sympathetic and parasympathetic nervous systems.** The sympathetic nervous system governs movement in the same way as the gas pedal in an automobile does. It activates the body's fight-or-flight response, providing it with more energy to respond to oncoming dangers. The parasympathetic nervous system acts as a brake. It promotes the "rest and digest" response, which calms the body when a danger has passed.

After receiving a distress signal from the amygdala, the hypothalamus activates the sympathetic nervous system by connecting with the adrenal glands through the autonomic nervous system. *In reaction, these glands produce the hormone epinephrine, sometimes known as adrenaline,* into the bloodstream. While adrenaline circulates throughout the body, many physiological changes occur. When the heart beats faster than normal, blood is pumped to the muscles, heart, and other vital organs. The heart rate and blood pressure rise. Furthermore, the person going through these changes tends to breathe faster. The tiny airways of the lungs are fairly open. In this method, the lungs may inhale as much oxygen as possible with each breath.

The brain obtains more oxygen, which increases alertness. Vision, hearing, and other senses improve. Meanwhile, epinephrine drives the body to release lipids and glucose from short-term storage areas. These nutrients flood the bloodstream, providing energy to the whole body.

Because all of these changes occur so quickly, no one sees them. The wiring is so effective that the amygdala and hypothalamus start the cascade before the brain's visual centers can fully understand what is going on. That explains why people may rush out of the path of an oncoming car without even thinking about it.

When the initial spike of epinephrine starts to fall, the hypothalamus activates the HPA axis, the second half of the stress response system. This network is made up of the hypothalamus, pituitary, and adrenal glands.

The sympathetic nervous system, sometimes known as the "gas pedal," is kept in check by the HPA axis through a series of hormone signals. If the brain continues to view something as dangerous, the hypothalamus creates **corticotropin-releasing hormone (CRH),** which travels to the pituitary gland and triggers the creation of **adrenocorticotropic hormone** (ACTH). This hormone visits the adrenal glands, causing them to create cortisol. As a consequence, the body is kept energetic and alert. Cortisol levels fall after the threat is passed. The "brake," or parasympathetic nervous system, then dampens the stress response.

Is stress a cause of Infertility?

Can my fertility be affected by stress? is one of the most often asked questions by those who are having difficulty conceiving. The goal of this book is to offer an overview of the studies supporting the influence of stress on reproductive outcomes. It also discusses our most current research in this area, which looks at the impact of the "stress hormone," cortisol, on IVF success.

In our fast-paced modern environment, stress may take many different forms and affect everyone at some time in our lives. Although the term "stress" has become a commonplace that we all use, it is not always well defined.

What exactly do we mean when we say we're "stressed"? Stress may be defined in a variety of ways, and what one person finds unpleasant may not be so for another. In general, "stress" is best defined as a pattern of physiological, behavioral, and cognitive responses to real or imagined stimuli (referred to as "stressors") that a person perceives as jeopardizing a goal or their welfare. Stress may last for a short or lengthy period of time. Acute stresses are brief and may originate from present demands and pressures or anticipated future requirements, such as making a public speech or being trapped in traffic on the way to work.

Chronic stressors are characterized by long-term strain, such as grief or coping with a medical condition such as infertility. Certain transient, short-term stress may even be useful to us, such as enhancing cognitive awareness and mobilizing energy to prepare us for "fight or flight." Chronic and long-term stress, on the other hand, may result in "allostatic load," which is a physiological wear and tear that can be hazardous to our health.

Two mechanisms primarily regulate the human stress response. These systems are known as the autonomic nervous system and the hypothalamic pituitary adrenal (HPA) axis. These two systems play a critical role in how our bodies respond to both short-term and long-term stress.

CORTISOL AND FERTILITY

Cortisol, a glucocorticoid hormone, is often referred to as a "biomarker of stress." Cortisol is secreted by the ***hypothalamus pituitary adrenal (HPA) axis,*** which is critical to the body's stress response. Cortisol is a hormone that affects physiological processes in the body such as metabolism, blood pressure, and reproduction. According to decades of research, the HPA axis is particularly vulnerable to stress, and greater cortisol levels caused by stress may have negative effects on a number of health outcomes. Massey et al. conducted a thorough review of over 1600 patients' worth of papers spanning 25 years that investigated how cortisol influences different IVF outcomes in 2014.

The researchers discovered 12 studies that investigated how cortisol affects pregnancy. The review discovered contradictory results on cortisol. In three studies, for example, greater cortisol levels were associated with an increased chance of pregnancy. According to four studies, high cortisol reduces the likelihood of conception. Five studies, however, were unable to find a link between cortisol and pregnancy. For a variety of reasons, the data supporting the impact of cortisol on fertility has been contradictory.

It is difficult to compare studies since most of them failed to account for recognized variables that influence cortisol levels, such as time of day (which is crucial because cortisol has a diurnal cycle). Second, the study looked at cortisol levels throughout different therapy periods. Despite the fact that IVF is a good clinical model for investigating how stress impacts reproductive outcomes, more than half of the studies (7/12) looked at cortisol levels after gonadotropin administration. Any observed links between HPA function and pregnancy are likely to have been obscured by gonadotropins, which have a considerable influence on the HPA axis.

These techniques have the disadvantage of only delivering a snapshot of hormone activity at a certain point in time, ranging from minutes to hours. Cortisol, on the other hand, is pulsatile, which means it fluctuates continually, similar to blood pressure. As a result, researchers have the issue of collecting between 3 and 9 samples throughout the day over a period of days in order to generate an accurate measurement of cortisol.

A relatively new approach for monitoring long-term cortisol levels, on the other hand, might offer huge promise for assessing how much stress impacts health and how cortisol affects fertility. Researchers can monitor cumulative long-term cortisol levels at up to 6-month intervals with a single non-invasive hair sample.

CORTISOL'S ROLE IN MENOPAUSE

Menopause is a natural stage of life, despite the fact that it only affects humans and a few marine creatures. As a woman enters her forties, the quantity of estrogen generated by her ovaries changes. They cease menstruation when this output reaches zero. The adrenal glands take over after the ovaries "retire," or cease generating sex hormones. They have reached menopause after a 12-month period without menstruation.

The four main hormones to monitor during menopause are as follows:

- **Estrogen**: When we think of menopause, we often think of estrogen, specifically estradiol (E2), the sex hormone that regulates the menstrual cycle. Perimenopause occurs when estrogen levels begin to fall, which usually occurs around the age of 45. (the commencement of the menopausal transition). However, estrogen is not simply vanishing at this time. It flies and tumbles like a roller coaster before crashing to the earth.

Many of the menopausal symptoms that women experience are caused by this, however the cause and effect relationship isn't always evident.

For example, both low and high estrogen levels are known to stress the body and influence cortisol levels. Cortisol levels must be balanced throughout our lives, but especially during menopause.

It's worth noting that many women will have an estrogen deficiency during the second half of their lives as a result of the dramatic increase in life expectancy. Estrogen insufficiency has been linked to degenerative illnesses of the cardiovascular, skeletal, and central nervous systems. Low estrogen levels may potentially exacerbate metabolic illness, leading to obesity, metabolic syndrome, type 2 diabetes, and even cancer (such as breast, colon, and liver cancer).

But there's another factor to consider: when estrogen levels fall, progesterone levels fall as well.

Prior to menopause, progesterone, often known as the "feel-good" hormone and the pregnancy hormone, was generated simultaneously with dehydroepiandrosterone (DHEA), which counteracts the effects of cortisol.

Progesterone levels often decline in perimenopausal women, reducing their capacity to cope with stress.

According to a recent research, women with higher levels of progesterone during the **perimenopause** reported significantly higher levels of life satisfaction, lower levels of perceived stress, and less depressive symptoms than those with lower levels. Progesterone may cause drowsiness and depression in certain women, as well as raise glucose levels, which might aggravate insulin resistance.

The stress hormone may be rising as progesterone falls.

The following information regarding cortisol is critical. But not simply the principal stress hormone. It regulates your sleep-wake cycle, blood sugar levels, energy metabolism, blood pressure, and many other things. When present in optimal proportions, it works quietly behind the scenes to maintain you in top form, with a slew of other hormones. Of course, cortisol is important in your stress reaction outside of your normal job. When you are under stress, whether mental or physical, your adrenal glands begin secreting extra cortisol to help you cope with the threat. In order to preserve energy, this may deactivate "non-essential" functionality.

That will help you survive in the short term. However, chronic cortisol imbalances may impair non-essential body activities such as digestion and reproduction, leading to a variety of medical problems. As a result, it is critical to monitor and regulate your cortisol levels in general. Menopausal women, in particular, wish to confirm their cortisol levels.

One effect of aging is a rise in cortisol levels. However, as previously mentioned, low estrogen levels may have an effect on cortisol levels. As a result, it should come as no surprise that the menopause is a stressful period, with various symptoms such as:

- Gaining weight and cravings for poor food
- Other sleep problems, such as insomnia
- A lack of sex desire and energy
- Aches and pains in addition
- Mood swings and sadness
- Hair and skin issues

Finally, both men and women manufacture testosterone in various physiological areas. This vital hormone, however, begins to drop with time, which has a significant influence on both sexes. In fact, many of the symptoms are comparable to those experienced by premenopausal women. For example, although depressive symptoms, fatigue, and sleep issues may worsen, sex drive and physical strength may diminish. Another study found that a higher **testosterone-to-estrogen** ratio at menopause was linked to depressive symptoms.

Our bodies adapt to the best of their ability throughout menopause. When our adrenal glands are constantly producing cortisol, they become less efficient in producing progesterone and other hormones. Our bodies will never put conception ahead of survival.

For example, 85 healthy women in their early menopause were studied (six months to five years postmenopause). In addition to lipid levels, the women's 24-hour urine cortisol levels and Greene Climacteric Scale scores (an early indication of menopausal symptoms) were evaluated. Finally, scientists established a link between all hormones. In other words, high cortisol levels have been associated with menopausal symptoms. According to the paper, *"increased cortisol is associated with known risk factors for cardiovascular disease, such as insulin resistance and a decreased (beneficial) HDL-cholesterol level."*

In actuality, an enzyme called 11betaHSD1 converts excess cortisol to cortisone, which is then stored in fat cells surrounding your organs. Cortisol, once reactivated and released, promotes binge eating, the accumulation of visceral fat, the development of diabetes, and may even cause depressed symptoms. This may exacerbate menopause's poor energy levels. High cortisol levels might promote low thyroid function, further depleting energy.

According to a different study, women with more frequent hot flashes had an unique cortisol pattern compared to those with less hot flashes. Those who awoke more often had lower cortisol levels on average. (They also had a tendency for higher cortisol levels before bed and lower diurnal volatility, but none of these patterns were statistically significant.) These anomalies may have an effect on both the quality of your sleep and your energy levels.

The good news is that by managing your cortisol levels, you may be able to reduce menopausal symptoms such as hot flashes, insomnia, and mood swings.

Acupuncture, phytoestrogens, or estrogen-progestin therapy were employed in one study to alleviate menopausal symptoms in 69 postmenopausal women (once a week). Researchers discovered that "a greater decrease in menopausal symptoms is associated with a larger drop in cortisol levels" when cortisol levels were tested. It is vital to study any possible ramifications of this finding for long-term consequences on women's health.

Despite the fact that the relationships between cortisol, estrogen, progesterone, testosterone, and other hormones in both men and women are complicated, one thing is certain: when one hormone is out of balance, others follow suit. Menopausal women face more than just psychological stress as a result of this complex domino effect. They are also physically tense.

You are stressed for a reason.
Progesterone and estrogen, which are terrific stress absorbers, are more likely to be present at optimal levels in women's bodies before menopause. When women's bodies degrade and perimenopausal hormone levels go wild, they have less defense against stress and high cortisol levels.

That may seem intimidating to a woman going through menopause. Despite the fact that premenopausal and menopausal women are commonly impacted by hormonal changes, the best ways to control them are usually not disclosed to them. Instead, they seek medical assistance and are prescribed antidepressants and anxiolytics. In the end, they often fail to address the underlying problem and have significant side effects.

RECOGNIZING THE RELATIONSHIP BETWEEN MENOPAUSAL SYMPTOMS AND STRESS-CORTISOL LEVELS.

Menopause is one of the most major physiological changes that women go through.

After all, it doesn't only impact and disrupt menstrual periods. It has the potential to disrupt some women's sleep cycles, metabolic functioning, cardiovascular health, and even mental well-being. Aside from the intermittent heat flashes, Some of these symptoms might continue for up to 10 years.

This might lead to conflict. Usually, changes to your body that seem sudden and random are. But what if we told you that these changes didn't have to be so drastic? What if women could go through menopause with greater assurance, less worry, and more preparedness?

That was one of the key reasons we decided to look into this endocrine problem. Paradigm is increasing human well being via scientific research on cortisol, the fundamental stress hormone. However, stress is just a minor factor in the cortisol equation.

Cortisol, you guessed it, has an effect on menopause. Indeed, the more we researched it and talked with our panel of experts, the more we realized how critical—and underappreciated—that stance is.

Contrary to popular belief, cortisol imbalances may play a part in the symptoms of menopause.